Nourishing Bites

A Meal Plan and Cookbook for Diabetics

Sara Mueller

Table of contents

Introduction

Thank you for visiting "Nourishing Bites: A Meal Plan and Cookbook for Diabetics" . We explore the realm of diabetes care via a tasty and nourishing lens in this all-inclusive book. You shouldn't have to give up flavor or enjoyment from your food because you have diabetes. With the correct information and resources, you can design a meal plan that satisfies your palate while also being good for your health.

Millions of individuals worldwide suffer from diabetes, which necessitates close monitoring to keep blood sugar levels steady. Eating a healthy diet is essential for controlling diabetes and enhancing general wellbeing. But it can be difficult to navigate the world of diabetic-friendly food, particularly when there are limitations and contradicting information available.

With this book, we hope to make meal planning easier for you and give you access to a variety of tasty and healthy recipes that are especially created for people with diabetes. We think eating healthfully should never be monotonous or constrictive. Rather, it ought to bring happiness, sustenance, and strength.

You'll discover a carefully chosen assortment of dishes in "Nourishing Bites" that are not only flavorful, textural, and varied, but also suitable for diabetics. We have everything you need, from filling dinners to hearty snacks, and from healthy breakfasts to delectable sweets. Every recipe has been meticulously created to satisfy the dietary needs of diabetics while also being a pleasure for everyone who share it at the table.

However, "Nourishing Bites" is not your average cookbook. You can also discover helpful information and advice about diabetes and its effects on nutrition within these pages. We'll go over the fundamentals of meal planning, show you how to successfully balance your macronutrients, and offer advice on how to shop for groceries and prepare meals.

We are aware that dealing with diabetes can be emotionally and physically taxing. For this reason, we've included chapters on how to manage stress, how to work out, and self-care techniques. We wish to assist you in every step of your quest for improved well-being and a happy life.

"Nourishing Bites" is designed to empower and encourage people with diabetes, regardless of how long they have been managing their condition or how recently they were diagnosed. We think eating healthfully should always be enjoyable and tasty rather than like a job. So let's get cooking and create some healthy snacks that will please your palate as well as your health requirements!

Recall that you are not by yourself. With "Nourishing Bites" as your guide, you'll be equipped with the information and skills necessary to embrace a creative, joyful, and confident diabetic existence. Prepare to turn your meals into something incredibly tasty and nutritious. One mouthful at a time, let's go on this path to a better, happier you.

Chapter 1

Understanding Nutrition and Diabetes: The Basics of Diabetes and it's impact on Nutrition

It's important to understand the basics of diabetes in order to appreciate how eating affects this condition. The hallmark of diabetes is elevated blood sugar levels, which arise from the body's incapacity to generate or efficiently utilize insulin, a hormone responsible for controlling blood sugar levels. The way that diet is impacted by this disturbance in insulin activity may be substantial.

Diabetes comes in various forms, the most prevalent being type 1 and type 2. An autoimmune condition known as type 1 diabetes occurs when the immune system unintentionally targets and kills the pancreatic cells that produce insulin. Insulin injections are necessary for people with type 1 diabetes to control their blood sugar levels.

Conversely, poor food choices, sedentary activity, and obesity are the main lifestyle variables linked to type 2 diabetes. It happens when the pancreas is unable to generate enough insulin to meet the body's needs, or when the body develops an immunity to insulin. A change in diet and exercise routine can help manage type 2 diabetes in many cases.

An essential component of managing diabetes is insulin. The body either doesn't make enough insulin or doesn't use it efficiently in people with diabetes. Insulin facilitates the movement of circulatory glucose into the cells, where it is utilised as an energy source. High blood sugar levels are caused by glucose building up in the bloodstream in the absence of enough insulin.

It's critical to comprehend how specific foods impact blood sugar levels when discussing diet and diabetes. Since carbohydrates are converted into glucose during digestion, they have the biggest effect on blood sugar. Simple carbohydrate foods include white bread, fizzy drinks, and sweets can spike blood sugar levels quickly.

Complex carbs, on the other hand, which are present in whole grains, legumes, and vegetables, are absorbed more gradually and raise blood sugar levels more gradually. For this reason, it's common advice for people with diabetes to include whole grains and high-fiber foods in their diet.

Blood sugar levels are not significantly impacted by fats or proteins. But it's crucial to go for lean protein sources like fish, chicken, and tofu as well as the healthy fats found in almonds, avocados, and olive oil. These options offer vital nutrients for general health in addition to helping with blood sugar regulation.

It's also critical to pay attention to meal timing and quantity sizes. Stable blood sugar levels can be achieved with eating regular, well-balanced meals throughout the day. Blood sugar spikes and falls can be avoided by distributing meals evenly and refraining from fasting for extended periods of time or overindulging.

People with diabetes can lower their risk of complications, maintain stable blood sugar levels, and live healthier lives by adopting educated dietary decisions.

Chapter 2

The Essentials of Diabetic Meal Planning

The foundational ideas of diabetic meal planning center on developing a customized, well-balanced strategy that meets individual requirements and preferences. People with diabetes can efficiently control their blood sugar levels and maintain general health by adhering to these guidelines.

Calculating one's daily carbohydrate consumption is a crucial part of meal planning for diabetes. Because they have the most effect on blood sugar levels, carbohydrates should be consumed in moderation throughout the day. The right amount of carbs to eat in each meal and snack can be determined by working with a certified dietitian, taking into account variables including age, activity level, and medication.

Another crucial idea is to provide a range of dietary categories. Lean proteins, high-fiber carbs, healthy fats, and an abundance of fruits and vegetables are all important components of a well-rounded diet plan. Proteins supply the necessary amino acids for maintaining and repairing muscles, and high-fiber carbs aid in blood sugar regulation and digestive well-being. Good fats supply vital nutrients and aid in satiety, and fruits and vegetables are rich in a variety of vitamins, minerals, and antioxidants.

Portion control is an additional essential concept. Blood sugar spikes can be avoided and calorie intake can be managed by keeping an eye on portion sizes. Estimating the right portion sizes can be aided by the use of measuring cups, food scales, or visual clues. Furthermore, being aware of your body's signals of hunger and fullness might help you avoid overindulging.

Adapting a meal plan to each person's unique requirements and tastes is essential for long-term success. Personal dietary preferences, cultural considerations, and lifestyle aspects should all be taken into account while preparing meals. Maintaining a healthy eating pattern and adhering to a meal plan can be facilitated by including foods that are enjoyable and satisfying.

It's crucial to take into account when to eat meals and snacks. Evenly spaced meals throughout the day can assist in preventing sharp swings in blood sugar levels and help keep them stable. If necessary, having snacks in between meals can help avoid hypoglycemia and hunger.

It's critical to monitor food glycemic index (GI) when developing a diabetic meal plan. Foods with a low GI have a slower, more gradual effect on blood sugar levels, whereas foods with a high GI can raise blood sugar levels quickly. Selecting foods low in glycemic index (GI), like legumes, whole grains, and non-starchy vegetables, can aid in promoting steady blood sugar regulation.

Last but not least, meal planning for diabetics should take into account personal objectives like controlling blood pressure or weight. Individuals can work toward achieving a well-rounded and comprehensive approach to their health by incorporating these goals into the overall plan.

For diabetics, meal planning should be adaptable, pleasurable, and long-lasting in order to support both blood sugar regulation and general wellbeing.

Chapter 3

Breakfast Delights: Energizing starts to your day

The most significant meal of the day is breakfast, so it's critical for people with diabetes to start the day off right with a variety of healthy breakfast options that help to keep blood sugar levels steady. Fortunately, there are lots of delectable recipes that can satisfy your hunger and supply you with the nutrients you need. Let's look at some stimulating breakfast options that will make your mornings more productive if you have diabetes.

Thick egg dishes are a great option for a breakfast that is diabetes-friendly. Eggs are a filling and nutrient-dense food because they are high in protein and healthy fats. You can enjoy a fluffy omelet filled with colorful vegetables like spinach, bell peppers, and onions. Another possibility is a veggie-packed frittata with mushrooms, zucchini, and cherry tomatoes. These egg dishes can be combined with a side of whole grain toast or a small quantity of cooked quinoa to add some fiber and complex carbohydrates to your meal.

Wholesome smoothies are another fantastic alternative to energize your mornings. Opt for low glycemic foods like berries, which have a smaller impact on blood sugar levels. Blend them with a source of protein such as

Greek yogurt or a plant-based protein powder. To improve the fiber content, add a handful of leafy greens like spinach or kale. You can also incorporate healthy fats by adding a tablespoon of nut butter or a sprinkle of chia seeds. These smoothies are not only refreshing but also contain a balanced combination of nutrients to keep you powered throughout the day.

Oatmeal is a staple breakfast choice that may be made diabetes-friendly with the correct additions. Choose steel-cut oats or old-fashioned rolled oats, which have a lower glycemic index compared to instant oats. Cook the oats in water or unsweetened almond milk and add a sprinkle of cinnamon for spice. Top your bowl of oatmeal with sliced almonds, chopped walnuts, or a tablespoon of ground flaxseeds for added texture and healthy fats. For natural sweetness and additional fiber, add a handful of berries or a sliced banana. This warm and cozy breakfast will keep you full and satisfied.

Greek yogurt parfait is another wonderful alternative that includes protein, healthy fats, and fiber. Layer Greek yogurt with low glycemic fruits like sliced strawberries or blueberries. Add a handful of crushed nuts or seeds for crunch and added nutrition. To improve the flavor, add a small quantity of honey or sprinkle some cinnamon on top. This parfait is not only physically stunning but also provides a balanced combination of macronutrients to start your day off well.

Remember, the key to a diabetes-friendly breakfast is to contain a solid dose of protein, healthy fats, and high-fiber carbohydrates. By including these items into your morning routine, you can have invigorating and enjoyable meals that keep your blood sugar levels constant. Try out a variety of recipes and ingredients to determine which ones work best for your dietary requirements and taste preferences. These breakfast treats can help you get motivated in the morning and prepare for a productive day.

Chapter 4

Wholesome Lunches: Fueling Your Afternoon

It's true that people with diabetes may find lunchtime challenging, but fear not! We will explore several delectable lunch ideas in this chapter that are not only healthful but also simple to make. These delicious choices will maintain stable blood sugar levels while providing you with sustained energy and satisfaction throughout the day. You'll find a variety of options that will tempt your taste buds, from colorful salads full of flavors to hearty soups that warm the spirit.

A vibrant salad is a great option for a meal that is suitable for those with diabetes. Begin with a bed of fresh, leafy greens, such as mixed lettuce or spinach. Next, add a variety of colorful veggies, like diced bell peppers, sliced cucumbers, grated carrots, and cherry tomatoes. Add grilled chicken breast, hard-boiled eggs, or legumes like black beans or chickpeas to boost the protein content. Add some seeds, such as pumpkin or sunflower, for crunch and good fats. For a last burst of flavor, dress your salad with a simple vinaigrette consisting of lemon juice, olive oil, and herbs.

Thick soups are a great alternative if you're craving something warm and satisfying. Choose homemade soups that are loaded with whole grains, lean meats, and a colorful assortment of vegetables. For example, you can make a delicious and nutritious vegetable and lentil soup by simmering lentils in a flavorful broth with a delightful combination of carrots, celery, onions, and bell peppers. To make it taste as good as it looks, add some flavorful herbs and spices like thyme, cumin, and turmeric. Serve your soup with some quinoa or whole grain bread on the side to round out the meal and add more complex carbohydrates and fiber.

Sandwiches and wraps are also delicious and easy options for a lunch that is suitable for people with diabetes. Choose bread or tortillas made from whole grains that are high in fiber. Stuff them with lean protein options such as turkey breast, grilled chicken, or even plant-based proteins like tofu or hummus. For a cool crunch, add lots of colorful and crunchy veggies like cucumbers, sliced tomatoes, and lettuce. For a creamy and nourishing touch, you can even add hummus or avocado spread. To complete the meal, these wraps and sandwiches can be served with some raw vegetables or a side salad.

Always remember to balance your intake of complex carbohydrates, protein, and healthy fats. You can make a wide range of delectable lunch options that not only satisfy your hunger but also offer vital nourishment by choosing a variety of nutrient-dense ingredients.

Chapter 5

Filling Snacks: Healthy Bits in Between

In fact, snacking can be very helpful in managing diabetes because it helps to keep blood sugar levels consistent throughout the day. In this chapter, we will delve into a variety of diabetic-friendly snacks that are not only satisfying but also brimming with essential nutrients. It's time to bid farewell to unhealthy choices and embrace a world of wholesome treats that will support your well-being.

When it comes to diabetic-friendly snacks, it's important to focus on nutrient-dense options that provide a balance of macronutrients - protein, healthy fats, and complex carbohydrates. One option is a handful of mixed nuts, such as almonds, walnuts, and cashews. Nuts are a fantastic source of healthy fats, fiber, and protein. They aid in blood sugar regulation in addition to maintaining a feeling of fullness and satisfaction. Just be mindful of portion sizes, as nuts are calorie-dense.

Fresh berries added to Greek yogurt makes for another delectable snack idea. Greek yogurt is a great option for people with diabetes because it is low in carbohydrates and high in protein. Top it off with a handful of antioxidant-rich berries like strawberries, blueberries, or raspberries. These fruits are rich in fiber, vitamins, and minerals and naturally sweet. This delightful combination of creamy yogurt and vibrant berries will leave you feeling nourished and satisfied.

Roasted chickpeas are a delicious and wholesome snack if you're craving something crunchy. Drain and rinse a can of chickpeas, then toss them with a drizzle of olive oil and a sprinkle of spices such as paprika, cumin, and garlic powder. Roast them in the oven until they turn crispy and golden. Chickpeas are a fantastic source of protein and fiber, making them an ideal snack for regulating blood sugar levels. Enjoy them on their own or as a topping for salads for an added crunch.

For a refreshing and hydrating snack, sliced vegetables with hummus are a perfect choice. Cut up an assortment of colorful vegetables like carrot sticks, cucumber slices, and bell pepper strips. Pair them with a generous serving of hummus, which is made from chickpeas and provides protein and fiber. The combination of crunchy vegetables and creamy hummus creates a satisfying snack that will keep you nourished and satisfied.

Snacking can be a beneficial part of managing diabetes when done right. By focusing on diabetic-friendly snacks that are nutrient-dense and balanced in macronutrients, you can satisfy your cravings while maintaining steady blood sugar levels. From mixed nuts to Greek yogurt with berries, roasted chickpeas, and sliced vegetables with hummus, there are plenty of wholesome treats to choose from. Embrace these nourishing morsels in

between meals and say hello to a healthier snacking
routine.

Chapter 6

Flavorful Dinners: Delicious and Diabetic-Friendly

Dinnertime should indeed be a time of excitement and culinary delight, even when following a diabetic meal plan. In this chapter, we will unveil a collection of exquisite and flavorful dinner recipes that will not compromise your health. From comforting stews to mouthwatering grilled dishes, you will have an array of options to choose from, ensuring that your taste buds are satisfied while still adhering to your diabetic needs.

One delectable option for a diabetic-friendly dinner is a comforting stew filled with robust flavors and wholesome ingredients. Consider preparing a hearty vegetable and bean stew, which combines an assortment of colorful vegetables like carrots, celery, onions, and bell peppers, with protein-packed beans such as kidney beans or chickpeas. Add aromatic herbs and spices like rosemary, thyme, and paprika to enhance the savory taste. Allow the stew to simmer slowly to bring out the rich flavors and make a warm and comforting supper that will leave you feeling full and pleased.

If you're in the mood for something grilled and filled with flavor, consider cooking a marinated chicken or fish meal. Create a marinade using a combination of herbs, spices, and citrus juices to infuse the meat with a burst of delectable taste. For chicken, a blend of garlic, lemon juice, and oregano can create a tangy and aromatic marinade. For fish, try a mix of lime juice, cilantro, and cumin for a zesty and refreshing flavor. Grill the marinated protein to perfection, and serve it alongside a colorful salad or a side of roasted vegetables for a well-rounded and satisfying dinner.

For those who crave the taste of international cuisine, a stir-fry can be a fantastic option. Stir-fries allow you to incorporate an array of vegetables, lean proteins, and flavorful sauces into one harmonious dish. Choose an assortment of colorful vegetables like bell peppers, broccoli, snap peas, and carrots, and pair them with lean proteins such as chicken or shrimp. Create a sauce using low-sodium soy sauce, ginger, garlic, and a bit of honey or a sugar replacement. Stir-fry the ingredients together until they are cooked to perfection, and serve it over a bed of cauliflower rice or whole grain noodles for a delicious and diabetes-friendly dinner.

Dinnertime should never be lacking in flavor or excitement. With the aid of these wonderful and diabetic-friendly dinner recipes, you can indulge in a variety of selections that will satisfy your taste buds while keeping your health in check. From comforting stews to mouthwatering grilled dishes and vibrant stir-fries, there are endless possibilities to explore. So, boost your dinnertime experience and taste the flavors of these delectable and diabetic-friendly recipes.

Chapter 7

Decadent Desserts: Sweet Treats without Compromising Health

Whoever suggested that folks with diabetes can't enjoy desserts definitely hasn't experienced the scrumptious treats we have in store for you! In this chapter, we will demonstrate a range of scrumptious dessert dishes that are not only low in sugar but also overflowing with flavor. Prepare to fulfill your sweet desire without compromising your health or experiencing any guilt. Get ready to indulge in these delectable delicacies that will leave you needing more.

One excellent choice for a diabetic-friendly dessert is a refreshing fruit salad. Choose a range of colorful and luscious fruits like berries, melons, citrus fruits, and kiwi. These fruits are naturally delicious and rich with critical vitamins and minerals. Add a sprinkling of chopped mint leaves or a splash of lemon juice to enhance the flavors. For an extra touch of indulgence, top your fruit salad with a dollop of Greek yogurt or a sprinkle of unsweetened coconut flakes. This dessert offers a healthy dose of antioxidants and fiber in addition to being light and delightful.

If you're craving something rich and creamy, you might want to try preparing a sugar-free cheesecake. Begin with a crust composed of melted butter combined with crumbled nuts or crushed graham crackers. Use a mixture of cream cheese, plain Greek yogurt, and an erythritol or stevia sugar alternative for the filling. For added taste, pour in a small amount of vanilla extract. Transfer the contents onto the crust and refrigerate until it solidifies. For a decadent and guilt-free dessert, top it with fresh berries or a drizzle of sugar-free chocolate sauce.

A thick and creamy chocolate avocado mousse is a must-try for chocolate fans. Smooth and creamy avocados are made when ripe avocados are blended with unsweetened cocoa powder, sugar replacement, a splash of almond milk, and a dash of salt. The cocoa powder offers a delicious chocolate flavor, and the avocados offer a creamy texture and good fats. To add a little additional opulence, top the mousse with a dollop of whipped cream or a sprinkle of crushed nuts after refrigerating it for a few hours.

You don't have to give up on savoring delectable treats because you have diabetes. These mouthwatering dessert recipes are suitable for those with diabetes, so you can satisfy your sweet taste without sacrificing your health. There are many options to fulfill every taste, ranging from rich chocolate avocado mousse to creamy cheesecakes and crisp fruit salads. You can have your

dessert and eat it too, even if you have diabetes, so let go
of any guilt and enjoy the richness of these delicious
sweets.

Chapter 8

Smart Grocery Shopping : Establishing a Diabetic Pantry

Creating a diabetic pantry is an essential part of eating a balanced, healthful diet. We'll walk you through the grocery store aisles in this chapter, offering advice on how to choose wisely and what to buy to help you on your diabetes meal planning adventure. Your meals will be tasty and nutritious if you keep your cupboard stocked with wholesome, diabetic-friendly options.

When choosing grains, choose for whole grains with a lower glycemic index and higher fiber content. Keep an eye out for foods like oats, brown rice, quinoa, and whole wheat pasta. These grains aid in blood sugar regulation and offer vital nutrients. If you want to bake, you might want to keep some whole grain flour on hand, like almond or whole wheat flour, which you might use in place of other flours in recipes.

A pantry that is suitable for diabetics must have protein. Select lean protein sources, such as tofu, skinless chicken breast, turkey, and fish. Due to their high fiber and protein content, dried or canned beans including lentils, black beans, and kidney beans are also fantastic choices. These adaptable components work well in a range of recipes, including stir-fries, salads, and soups.

It is crucial to concentrate on healthy options when it comes to fats. Choose heart-healthy fat-containing oils like coconut, avocado, or olive oil. Rich in protein, fiber, and good fats, nuts and seeds like flaxseeds, chia seeds, and walnuts are excellent additions to your pantry. They can be eaten as a snack or added to salads and yogurt as a topping.

There are sugar substitutes available in the sweetener market that can be used sparingly. Natural sugar substitutes like erythritol, stevia, and monk fruit extract can sweeten your dishes without significantly raising blood sugar levels. These sweeteners can be used in baking or to sweeten drinks; they come in granulated or liquid form.

Select low-sodium options for canned goods whenever possible. Seek for canned veggies that haven't had any added sugars or salt added, like diced tomatoes, green beans, or corn. Canary fish, like salmon or tuna, is a great way to get omega-3 fatty acids and can be added to salads or sandwiches.

Last but not least, remember to stock your pantry with a range of herbs, spices, and sauces. Your meals can benefit from the depth and flavor that these ingredients can provide without overusing sugar or salt. Garlic powder, onion powder, low-sodium soy sauce, vinegar, mustard, and dried herbs like oregano and basil are popular options.

Creating a pantry that is suitable for people with diabetes is a critical first step in meal planning success. Your pantry can be filled with wholesome options that help you achieve your health goals if you make wise decisions and choose the right ingredients. Your ability to prepare tasty and diabetes-friendly meals will be enhanced by having a well-stocked pantry that includes whole grains, lean proteins, healthy fats, sugar replacements, and an assortment of herbs and spices. So let's start shopping wisely for groceries and stock our diabetic pantry to lay the groundwork for a fulfilling and healthful mealtime.

Chapter 9

Mastering Portion Control: Keeping Carbs, Proteins, and Fats in Check

Welcome to the chapter on mastering portion management for diabetics! When it comes to controlling your diabetes, portion management is a critical ability to learn. By understanding how to negotiate portion sizes and balance your macronutrients properly, you can maintain stable blood sugar levels and produce meals that are both healthy and satisfying.

The first step in mastering portion management is to become familiar with acceptable serving sizes for different food groups. Carbohydrates, proteins, and fats are the three macronutrients that make up our meals. Carbohydrates have the most significant impact on blood sugar levels, therefore it's crucial to be cautious of the quantity consumed. Aim for roughly 45-60 grams of carbohydrates per meal, but note that this may vary depending on your particular needs and suggestions from your healthcare professional.

Proteins are crucial for maintaining muscular mass and generating a sensation of fullness. When portioning proteins, aim for a serving size of roughly 3-4 ounces per meal. This can be roughly similar to the size of a deck of cards or the palm of your hand. Opt for lean sources of protein such as skinless chicken, turkey, fish, tofu, or lentils. These selections offer high-quality nourishment without excessive fat or carbohydrates.

Fats are an important part of a balanced diet, but they are also calorie-dense. It is important to portion fats carefully, considering the amount that is really consumed. Nuts, seeds, avocados, and olive oil are good sources of healthy fats that are good for your heart and general health. For each meal, try to include one to two teaspoons of healthy fats, depending on your dietary objectives and specific needs.

Apart from weighing portion sizes, it's crucial to take into account the overall composition of your meals. Make an effort to arrange your food such that the proportions of fats, proteins, and carbohydrates are all in harmony. This will guarantee that you're getting a range of vital nutrients, assist maintain stable blood sugar levels, and provide you long-lasting energy. Remember to add a lot of vibrant veggies to your meals as well. They can help you feel full without adding too many calories or carbohydrates because they are high in fiber, vitamins, and minerals.

It takes practice to become proficient at controlling portion sizes and achieving a healthy macronutrient balance. Gaining an intuitive understanding of portion proportions may require some time and practice, but the work is well worth it. Always remember that working with a registered dietitian or other healthcare professional is always advantageous since they can offer individualized advice and help in adjusting portion sizes and the balance of macronutrients to meet your unique needs. You can take charge of your diabetes care and prepare wholesome, tasty meals by learning how to reduce your portion sizes. Together, let's take the path towards portion control and prepare meals that are well-balanced and promote your overall health and wellbeing.

Chapter 10

Organizing Your Meals for Success: Conserving Time and Energy

Greetings and welcome to the chapter on diabetic meal preparation for success! For many people, including those who manage diabetes, meal preparation really does make a big difference. You can ensure that you always have scrumptious and nourishing options available while also saving a ton of time and effort by planning and preparing your meals ahead of time.

Simplifying your cooking process is one of the main advantages of meal prep. You can spend a few hours on a chosen day prepping your meals for the week rather than spending hours in the kitchen every day. This lessens the stress of having to decide what to cook every day and saves time as well. When your meals are prepared and ready to eat, you can concentrate on eating well and looking after yourself.

Achieving success in meal prep requires careful planning. Make a meal plan that suits your dietary requirements and preferences first. Think about including a range of nutrient-dense foods, such as whole grains, lean proteins, an abundance of fruits and vegetables, and healthy fats. By doing this, you can make sure that your meals are nutritious and well-balanced,

supporting both the management of your diabetes and
your general health.

After you've decided on your menu, create a thorough
grocery list and shop appropriately. You'll save time and
avoid errands at the last minute if you have all the
ingredients on hand. To save money and cut down on
food waste, think about buying products in bulk or
opting for frozen options. Purchasing high-quality food
storage containers will also assist in maintaining the
freshness and accessibility of your prepared meals
throughout the workweek.

When it comes time to meal prep, begin by cleaning,
chopping, and dividing up your ingredients. This not
only facilitates speedy meal preparation during the
week, but it also saves time. Cook your proteins, such as
chicken, fish, or tofu, in larger batches and portion them
out into individual containers. Similarly, you can
prepare grains, like quinoa or brown rice, and store
them separately for easy meal assembly.

Don't forget about snacks and on-the-go options.
Prepping healthy snacks, such as cut-up vegetables, fruit
cups, or homemade energy balls, can help you avoid
reaching for less nutritious choices when hunger strikes.
Having these snacks readily available can be a lifesaver,
especially when you're on the go or in need of a quick
pick-me-up.

To keep your meals interesting and flavorful, explore different recipes and flavors. Experiment with spices, herbs, and marinades to add variety and enhance the taste of your meals. There are numerous resources available, including cookbooks and online recipe databases, that offer diabetic-friendly meal prep ideas and inspiration.

By dedicating a little time each week to meal prepping, you can save time and effort while ensuring that you have nourishing meals at your fingertips. Embrace the benefits of meal prepping, and enjoy the convenience of having delicious and nutritious creations waiting for you. So, let's dive into the world of meal prepping and discover how it can help you on your journey to managing diabetes and living a healthy, balanced life.

Chapter 11

Dining Out with Diabetes: Making Wise Choices

Welcome to the chapter on dining out with diabetes! Eating out at restaurants can be a wonderful experience, and having diabetes shouldn't hold you back from enjoying delicious meals. With the correct knowledge and tactics, you can make intelligent decisions that assist your blood sugar management without compromising taste or enjoyment.

When dining out, one of the first stages is to choose the right restaurant. Look for establishments that offer a choice of healthful options and are willing to accommodate unique dietary demands. Many restaurants now give nutritional information on their menus or websites, which can be a great resource for making educated choices. Additionally, consider exploring ethnic cuisines like Mediterranean or Asian, as they typically offer delectable dishes that are high in veggies, lean proteins, and healthy fats.

Navigating the menu is another key component of dining out with diabetes. Start by checking the menu for phrases that imply healthier selections, such as grilled, baked, or steamed. Look for dishes that incorporate lean proteins like chicken, fish, or tofu, and go for nutritious grains and veggies as side dishes. Avoid menu items that are labeled as fried, breaded, or creamy, as these likely to be higher in unhealthy fats and carbohydrates.

Portion control is vital for treating diabetes, and this applies to dining out as well. Many restaurants often serve large portions that can exceed your recommended intake of calories and carbohydrates. Consider splitting a meal with a dining partner or asking for a half portion. If neither of these solutions is practicable, ask for a to-go container when your food arrives and portion out a smaller piece before you start eating. This manner, you can enjoy your meal while being aware of portion sizes.

Don't be scared to ask questions or make unique requests when dining out. Most restaurants are willing to accommodate dietary demands and can give changes to fit your preferences. For example, you can order dressings or sauces on the side, substitute high-carbohydrate sides with vegetables, or ask for grilled alternatives instead of fried. Communicating your demands with the waitstaff or chef can assist ensure that your meal is served in a way that corresponds with your dietary goals.

Lastly, try to listen to your body and eat mindfully when dining out. Pay attention to your hunger and fullness cues, and eat at a slower pace to allow your brain to recognize when you're satisfied. Eating slowly and watching your portion sizes can assist avoid overindulging because it's easy to be swept up in the social aspect of eating out.

Eating out may be a pleasant and diabetes-friendly experience if you have the correct information and techniques. You may enjoy eating out and manage your blood sugar while making informed decisions by picking the proper restaurant, navigating the menu, exercising portion control, making specific requests, and eating mindfully. So feel free to enjoy eating out with confidence while maintaining a healthy diabetes regimen.

Chapter 12

Managing Stress and Emotional Eating

We all experience stress from time to time, and it can negatively impact our general health, particularly for those who are managing diabetes. Stress not only affects blood sugar levels but also triggers emotional eating as a coping strategy. It is essential to comprehend the relationship between stress, diabetes, and emotional eating in order to create good coping mechanisms for these conditions.

Hormones that can raise blood sugar levels are released when under stress. For those who have diabetes, this may be troublesome since it may be harder to have stable blood sugar management. Stress can also influence appetite regulation, interfere with sleep cycles, and lead to unhealthy habits like emotional eating. The propensity to eat in response to feelings rather than actual hunger is known as emotional eating, and it frequently results in the ingestion of comfort foods that are high in calories and may not be appropriate for a diabetic's diet.

It is crucial to have appropriate coping techniques in order to prevent emotional eating and handle stress. Frequent exercise is one of the best ways. In addition to lowering stress levels, exercise can enhance insulin sensitivity and enhance general wellbeing. Walking, yoga, and swimming are a few exercises that can help reduce stress and give you a healthy way to release your feelings.

Creating effective stress-reduction strategies is a crucial part of controlling stress and emotional eating. Methods like mindfulness exercises, meditation, or deep breathing exercises can assist lower stress and promote mental calmness. Choosing enjoyable and soothing hobbies, like reading, listening to music, or going on a nature walk, can also help with stress management and stop emotional eating.

Creating a network of support is essential for stress management and emotional eating. Make an effort to connect with loved ones, friends, or a support group who may provide understanding and assistance during trying times. Finding healthy coping mechanisms for stress can be facilitated by talking to others about your feelings and worries.

Managing emotional eating requires cultivating an intuitive and aware relationship with food. Eating mindfully entails observing your body's hunger signals, taking your time, and enjoying every bite. It also entails being conscious of the emotional triggers that could result in unhealthful eating habits. You can choose when and what to eat more thoughtfully if you know the difference between emotional and physical hunger.

For diabetics, controlling stress and emotional eating is essential. You can effectively manage your stress levels by learning healthy coping mechanisms, such as regular exercise, stress management techniques, and creating a support network. Furthermore, emotional eating can be avoided and general wellbeing can be supported by engaging in mindful eating and cultivating an intuitive relationship with food. Recall that stress management encompasses more than just controlling your blood sugar levels; it also entails looking after your general health and wellbeing.

Chapter 13

Staying Active and fit: Exercise tips for Diabetics

Regular exercise is a key component of managing diabetes and improving overall health. Engaging in physical activity not only helps control blood sugar levels but also contributes to weight management, improves cardiovascular health, boosts mood, and enhances overall well-being. In this chapter, we will explore exercise tips and routines specifically tailored for individuals with diabetes.

Cardiovascular exercises, such as walking, jogging, cycling, or swimming, are excellent choices for managing diabetes. Aim for at least 150 minutes of moderate-intensity aerobic activity per week, spread out over several days. If you're just starting out, begin with shorter sessions and gradually increase the duration and intensity as your fitness level improves. Find activities that you enjoy and that are accessible to you, whether it's taking a brisk walk in your neighborhood or joining a dance class. Remember to monitor your blood sugar levels before, during, and after exercise, and adjust your medication or food intake accordingly.

In addition to cardiovascular exercise, incorporating strength training into your routine is highly beneficial for individuals with diabetes. Strength training helps build muscle mass, improves insulin sensitivity, and aids in weight management. Include exercises that target major muscle groups, such as squats, lunges, push-ups, and rows. Start with lighter weights or resistance bands and gradually increase the resistance as you become stronger. Aim for two to three strength training sessions per week, allowing at least 48 hours of rest between sessions to allow your muscles to recover and rebuild.

Flexibility exercises are also important for maintaining joint mobility and preventing injuries. Incorporate stretching exercises into your routine, focusing on major muscle groups like the hamstrings, quadriceps, and shoulders. Yoga and Pilates are excellent options for improving flexibility, balance, and overall body awareness. Remember to warm up before any exercise session and cool down afterward to prevent muscle soreness and promote recovery.

It's essential to listen to your body when engaging in physical activity. Pay attention to any signs of discomfort, pain, or dizziness, and adjust your intensity or seek medical advice if needed. Stay hydrated during your workouts by drinking water regularly, and always carry a source of fast-acting carbohydrates, like glucose tablets or fruit juice, in case of low blood sugar.

If you're new to exercise or have any underlying health conditions, it's always a good idea to consult with your healthcare team before starting a new fitness regimen.

They can provide guidance and recommendations based on your specific needs and health status.

Remember, staying active and fit is a lifelong journey. Find activities that you enjoy and make them a regular part of your routine. Consistency is key, so aim for a balance of cardiovascular exercise, strength training, and flexibility exercises. By staying active, you can effectively manage your diabetes, improve your overall health, and enjoy the countless benefits that regular exercise brings. So, lace up your sneakers, grab your resistance bands, and embark on a journey to a healthier, fitter you!

Chapter 14

Diabetic-Friendly Beverages: Quenching Your Thirst

Staying hydrated is crucial for everyone, and it's particularly important for individuals with diabetes. However, it can be challenging to find beverage options that are both flavorful and won't spike your blood sugar levels. In this chapter, we'll explore a variety of refreshing and diabetic-friendly options to quench your thirst.

One of the simplest and healthiest beverage options is infused water. Infusing water with fruits, vegetables, or herbs adds flavor without adding unnecessary sugars or calories. Try adding slices of citrus fruits like lemon, lime, or orange, along with a sprig of mint or a few cucumber slices, to a pitcher of water. Let it sit in the refrigerator for a few hours to allow the flavors to infuse. This natural infusion provides a refreshing and hydrating drink without any added sugars.

Herbal teas are another great option for diabetics. Unlike traditional teas that contain caffeine, herbal teas are made from a variety of plants and do not contain any caffeine. Choose herbal teas like chamomile, peppermint, or hibiscus, which not only provide hydration but also offer potential health benefits. These teas can be enjoyed hot or cold, depending on your preference, and can be sweetened with a sugar substitute if desired.

If you're looking for something a bit more exciting, consider making sugar-free mocktails. Mocktails are non-alcoholic cocktails that can be just as tasty and refreshing as their alcoholic counterparts. Start by picking a sugar-free foundation, such as diet soda, sparkling water, or unsweetened fruit juice. Then, add fresh fruits, herbs, or sugar-free flavorings to enhance the taste. For example, you may create a delightful mojito mocktail by muddling fresh mint leaves, lime juice, and a sugar alternative, and then topping it off with sparkling water. Get creative and experiment with different mixtures to find your favorite diabetic-friendly mocktail.

Another choice for diabetic-friendly beverages is unsweetened iced tea. Brew a pot of your favorite tea, such as black, green, or herbal, and let it cool before pouring it over ice. You can add a squeeze of lemon or a few drops of liquid sugar substitute to enhance the flavor without adding any additional sugar. This thirst-quenching solution delivers a selection of tastes to suit diverse preferences while avoiding the extra sugars found in pre-sweetened iced teas.

When picking beverages, it's crucial to check labels and be cautious of the sugar content. Avoid sugary sodas, fruit juices, and energy drinks, as these can cause a rapid spike in blood sugar levels. Opt for sugar-free or diet versions of your favorite drinks, or choose liquids that are naturally low in sugar, such as water or unsweetened tea.

There are many of diabetic-friendly beverage options to keep you refreshed and hydrated without damaging your blood sugar levels. Experiment with infused water, herbal teas, sugar-free mocktails, and unsweetened iced tea to find the tastes that appeal to you. By making attentive decisions and exploring creative alternatives, you can enjoy a variety of delicious and diabetic-friendly beverages that will quench your thirst and promote your overall well-being. Let's toast to being hydrated and well!

Chapter 15

Living Well with Diabetes: Support, Self-care, and Beyond

To ensure a happy and healthy life, it is crucial to prioritize support and self-care in the long-term management of diabetes. We'll discuss the value of seeking support in this chapter, including through professional assistance and participation in support groups. We'll also talk about how important self-care routines are to properly managing diabetes.

The support of others who have experienced what they are going through is one of the most important resources for people with diabetes. Getting involved in a support group can help you connect with people who have gone through similar things and build a sense of community. A safe place to express emotions, pose inquiries, and gain knowledge from one another is provided by support groups. Local support groups can be located in your area, or you can look into online communities to interact with people worldwide. Recall that you are not alone in your diabetes journey, and that getting help can have a big impact on your general health.

For diabetes to be properly managed, getting professional assistance is essential in addition to attending support groups. Your medical team, which consists of physicians, nurses, dietitians, and diabetes educators, can offer direction, instruction, and customized treatment regimens. Making routine appointments with your healthcare team will help you stay on top of your diabetes management and will allow you to ask any questions or address any concerns you may have. They can also assist you in monitoring your progress, helping you set reasonable goals, and modifying your treatment plan as needed.

Practicing self-care is essential to having a healthy diabetes lifestyle. Taking care of yourself is crucial for your general well-being, as managing diabetes can be mentally and emotionally taxing. Prioritizing self-care activities such as getting enough sleep, engaging in regular physical activity, and practicing stress management techniques can help you maintain a healthy lifestyle. It's also important to make time for activities that bring you joy and relaxation, whether it's reading a book, listening to music, practicing a hobby, or spending time with loved ones. Remember, taking care of yourself is not selfish but necessary for managing your diabetes effectively.

Additionally, monitoring your blood sugar levels regularly, taking your prescribed medications, and following a diabetes-friendly diet are crucial aspects of self-care. This includes monitoring your carbohydrate intake, choosing nutrient-dense foods, and practicing portion control. Working with a registered dietitian can provide you with personalized guidance and support in developing a diabetes-friendly meal plan that suits your individual needs and preferences.

Finally, seeking support, both through support groups and professional help, is essential for individuals living with diabetes. Surrounding yourself with a supportive community and seeking guidance from healthcare professionals can provide valuable resources and assistance in managing your diabetes effectively. Additionally, prioritizing self-care practices, such as engaging in regular physical activity, practicing stress management techniques, and taking care of your mental and emotional well-being, is crucial for living a fulfilling life while managing diabetes. Remember, you have the power to live well with diabetes and thrive in all aspects of your life.

Conclusion

In conclusion, "Nourishing Bites: A Meal Plan and Cookbook for Diabetics" offers a comprehensive guide to managing diabetes through healthy eating. Throughout this book, we have explored the fundamentals of diabetes management, including the importance of balanced nutrition, portion control, and mindful eating. We have offered a choice of delicious and healthy meals that cater to the special dietary demands of those with diabetes.

By following the meal plan and adopting the recipes in this book into your daily routine, you can take control of your diabetes and enhance your general well-being. The recipes are designed to be delectable, gratifying, and easy to prepare, making healthy eating both pleasurable and accessible. From breakfast alternatives to main courses, snacks, and desserts, we have supplied a varied range of recipes that meet various tastes and dietary needs.

Additionally, we have dug into crucial issues such as understanding carbs, managing blood sugar levels, and making smart eating choices. The meal plan and cookbook serve as a significant tool for individuals with diabetes, empowering them to make healthier food choices, create sustainable eating habits, and reach their health goals.

It is crucial to remember that controlling diabetes is a lifelong process, and there may be hurdles along the road. However, with the knowledge and resources presented in this book, you have the tools to overcome those hurdles and create great changes in your life. Remember to consult with your healthcare team for specialized advice and guidance.

Ultimately, "Nourishing Bites: A Meal Plan and Cookbook for Diabetics" is more than just a compilation of recipes. It is a guide to having a balanced, satisfying, and fulfilling life with diabetes. By nourishing your body with healthful and delicious meals, you are playing an active role in your health and well-being. With determination, mindfulness, and the help of your healthcare team, you may successfully manage your diabetes and maintain a bright and healthy life.

Thank you for joining us on our journey towards greater health through nourishing bites. May this book serve as a great resource and companion in your quest for a fulfilling life with diabetes. Cheers to excellent health and wonderful meals!

www.ingramcontent.com/pod-product-compliance
Lightning Source LLC
Chambersburg PA
CBHW070736260726
48660CB00007B/2870